G.M.O. Free Diet

How to stay healthy by identifying and avoiding dangerous foods

Table of Contents

Introduction

I want to thank you and congratulate you for reading this book, "G.M.O. Free Diet: How to stay healthy by identifying and avoiding dangerous foods".

GMO stands for Genetically Modified Organism. It means the original DNA of a plant or animal has been changed under laboratory conditions.

Many countries have banned these controversial foods all over the world including Australia, Japan, and most of Europe. They have been labeled as potentially toxic and dangerous to consume. Despite this, these foods are everywhere, especially in the United States.

This book contains steps and strategies on how you can identify both common and uncommon GMO foods and where they may be hidden in common processed food ingredients. The resources in this book will empower you to create a diet free from GMO ingredients.

It is also the intent of this book to expose the many "healthy" everyday items and brands that contain genetically modified ingredients. Some of them may surprise you.

In the United States, over 75% of all food contains GMO's. Currently there are no regulations requiring GMO foods to be labeled and food advertised as organic or healthy is often loaded with ingredients that are in fact genetically modified.

We all know diets can be challenging and when you're working hard to stay healthy you want to give your body maximum nutrition and avoid potentially harmful ingredients. This is why it is critical that you are aware of the potential sources of GMO contamination.

These genetically modified foods are not mandatory to consume. We all have the power of choosing what we are putting in our bodies. Giving this power away to corporations such as Monsanto, could be a fatal mistake. These companies spend lots of money to keep us unaware of the potential dangers in the "food" they "create".

No matter what type of diet you subscribe to, GMO foods are out there. If you are committed to staying healthy and fit, it is my hope that the information contained in this book will help you make intelligent decisions about the food you eat.

Thanks again for reading this book, I hope you enjoy it!

Chapter 1

What are GMO Foods?

The first action step for eating a GMO Free Diet is to know how and why these "foods" came into existence in the first place. This step is essential to making an informed decision on whether or not you choose to consume these products.

Genetically Modified Organisms, also known as GMOs, are plants or animals created through gene splicing techniques (also called genetic engineering, or GE). This technology is experimental and merges DNA from different species, creating unstable combinations of plant, animal, bacterial and viral genes that cannot occur in nature or in traditional crossbreeding.

There are many reasons given to the public for altering our food through genetic engineering. They include, but are not limited to: faster growth, resistance to pathogens (including pesticides) and insects, production of extra nutrients, and decreasing the cost of production. We will later discover the true intention of GMO's.

The process of genetically engineering foods is often justified by comparing it to traditional crossbreeding of foods, but in fact the two processes are very different. One process being completely natural, while the other being anything but. When it comes to diet and the body, the natural route has proven itself to be the tried and true path to optimum health.

Let's examine the process in a little more detail.

Genetic engineering crosses species by introducing genes that are absolutely foreign. An example of GE would be introducing a gene from a fish into a tomato or DNA from bacteria into corn. Traditional crossbreeding is always done between same or similar species. For instance, a mildew-resistant pea and a high-yield pea can be crossed naturally.

GE takes place in a laboratory whereas traditional crossbreeding occurs naturally on Earth. It is an artificial placement of a gene into another species under laboratory conditions. Traditional crossbreeding is free of manipulation and is simply the choosing of certain parents for mating: a natural combination of substances.

Simply speaking, traditional crossbreeding is dependent upon the natural reproductive process, while genetic engineering uses artificial parts of genetic material introduced into plant and animal cells using chemical, mechanical or bacterial methods. GE can result in an unpredictable substance that can be allergenic or even toxic.

The field of genetically modified foods is a new one comparatively speaking. The short term effects of these foods on the body are disturbing enough alone, not to mention the long term consequences that will most likely not be seen for years to come.

These are experimental foods created in a lab. Flounder fish are being fused with tomatoes, moth genes are being fused with potatoes, and firefly genes are being fused with corn. They have even made crops that produce their own insecticide. Sounds delicious right?

Unfortunately that is not all. In order for these combinations to take place, scientists use bacteria and viruses to invade the cell of a plant. Since a healthy cell will automatically reject foreign material, a method was created using soil bacteria that cause tumors in plants.

The bacteria act as a transportation system to deliver the altered DNA material into the nucleus of a cell.

Another method uses what is referred to as a gene gun. This device shoots gold particles coated with altered DNA material into plant cells.

The next step for either of these methods is to use a virus. Once inside the nucleus the altered genetic material spreads to all the other cells of a plant using a virus gene, often the cauliflower mosaic virus.

Tumors in plants, and bacteria together with viruses in food does not really sound like progress in my opinion. What authority could convince someone that these foods are safe? For me there isn't one.

This cocktail of bacteria and viruses often result in genetic mutations. What are the consequences of ingesting these mutated foods over a period of time? The ability to change the genetic makeup of a mammal with foods that have been engineered with a virus is something to stop and think about.

The United States currently does not require biotechnology companies to do premarket safety testing including allergen testing. Independent studies have actually shown these foods to cause an increase in weight gain. In 2012 a paper by Eric Seralini, a researcher at the University of Caen in France, found a GM corn diet led to cancer in rats.

There are plenty of diseases in the world today that are linked to diet. Today it is common knowledge what eating habits make us fat, and what eating habits promote energy and overall health. By eating genetically modified foods one has to wonder what the consequences will be.

 Now that some of the facts are out of the way and we understand these foods are obviously experimental, we can make a conscious decision whether or not we want to be experimented on.

Whether you are skeptical of GMO foods or believe that they are a beneficial scientific advancement, the fact remains there is no guarantee that GMO foods will not do serious damage to the body over time. No proven track record can be given because one simply does not exist.

In order to be confident that your healthy eating habits and physical exercise are going to actually pay off for all the hard work you put in, common sense would suggest avoiding these experimental foods all together.

After all, the natural cycles of Earth have been abundantly supplying perfectly designed nourishment for thousands and thousands of years. If it's not broke why fix it? The interest large companies have in this technology will become apparent in the next chapter.

There is no good reason a food company could give for wanting to use these genetically altered ingredients. Whether these companies are full of good intentions or have a sinister goal, the fact remains that they are still experimental. In my opinion, and the opinion of many nations around the world, these foods should not be consumed.

Experiments, by definition, have unknown outcomes. However, the outcome of eating healthy foods designed by nature is well known and it is how people have sustained themselves on this planet for thousands of years.

Chapter 2

The Monsanto Corporation

The story of what GMO foods are would not be complete without mentioning the Monsanto Corporation. They are the architects of many GMO crops.

Here is a short story of how genetically modified crops came into being.

The Monsanto Corporation is well known for its chemical pesticide brand Roundup but originally they were known for the chemical known as Agent Orange. For those who don't know, Agent Orange was used in the Vietnam War as a form of chemical warfare, and Monsanto was contracted by the US Department of Defense to produce this chemical.

Their "success" in the chemical business then led to their brand of herbicide called Roundup. In the year 2000 the patent on their popular Roundup brand was due to expire. In an effort to prolong their patent, Monsanto created Roundup Ready crops. These crops were genetically altered using the process described in the previous chapter and designed for the specific purpose of being tolerant to Roundup herbicide treatments.

This also allowed Monsanto to be awarded patents on these new strains of genetically modified crops. Upon purchasing these genetically modified seeds, a farmer enters into a contract with Monsanto to purchase the Roundup chemical as well.

In addition, the farmer is only licensing the seed for one year. A farmer is no longer allowed to collect their own seeds as farmers have done for thousands of years. Not only are the foods being grown from these seeds sprayed with toxic chemicals, but as previously discussed they are full of genetic mutations.

The business plan of most large corporate businesses is profit. Monsanto is no different and their goal is to own the food supply of the entire Earth with their patented products.

There have been several lawsuits initiated by Monsanto to shut down farms of farmers that were found growing these patented crops. These farmers were unaware the patented crops were growing on their land. Pollen from other farms can travel for hundreds of miles carried by the wind, and may cross pollinate with natural strains. This creates a strain that now has the altered genetic material embedded in the plants DNA.

The idea of cross pollination is frightening. This means that over time, all foods will have some level of the patented, genetically modified DNA embedded into them. This would make them the property of the corporation and is the endgame for Monsanto, granting them legal ownership of the food supply on Earth.

Seeds can also be carried by birds or blown in from neighboring farms leaving a farmer with little to no control over the situation

The process of modifying genetic material in plants causes countless mutations to the DNA and can cause allergens, toxins, and many other dangerous and harmful effects. These accusations are dismissed by Monsanto; however they are being discovered and exposed by independent researchers and scientists.

So in short the chemical warfare business was slow and this corporation decided to go into the food and agriculture business. Not a very natural progression in my opinion.

Add to this the fact that many Monsanto executives are revolving door seat holders in government entities such as the FDA, and EPA.

For instance, Michael Taylor, the deputy commissioner for the FDA (Food and Drug Administration) wrote the guidelines for labeling genetically engineered bovine growth hormone. This hormone is injected into cows to make them produce more milk. The same Michael Taylor at the time was a lawyer for the Monsanto Corporation. Later he became Vice President of Monsanto. Recently President Obama appointed this same man as Senior Advisor to the FDA.

There are dozens of instances where government officials with the authority to write new policy, also work for the Monsanto Corporation.

Here are just a few more examples: Margaret Miller, top Monsanto scientist and also Deputy Director of the FDA in the 1990's.

Toby Moffett is a Monsanto consultant and US Congressman.

Dennis DeConcini is Monsanto legal counsel and a US Senator.

Donald Rumsfeld was the previous CEO of Searle (a company that merged with Monsanto). While he held this position he was able to get aspartame legalized. This same man was appointed to Secretary of Defense in 1975 and again in the year 2000.

The list goes on and on.

The Monsanto Corporation was asked by Arthur Anderson, (a consultant that worked with Monsanto in the 1990's and later with Enron), to describe their ideal business position in 20 years. Monsanto executives described a world where 100% of the world's seeds were genetically modified, patented, and owned by them. They then developed a strategy to work backwards from that goal to achieve their mission.

Simply put, you would no longer be able to grow your own food without consent from the patent holder, the Monsanto Corporation. This obviously cannot be allowed to happen.

So to recap, a company involved in chemical warfare in the previous century has decided to replace the billions of years of evolution and perfect design that natural foods have to offer, with their new patented product. Common sense suggests this is very wrong on many levels. It is an experiment that I hope you, the reader of this book, will not only to refuse to take part in, but help put a stop to.

An entire book could be written on Monsanto and their tactics. Many books and documentaries have indeed been created around this controversial corporation. Take a look in the back of this book for suggested reading and documentaries concerning Monsanto.

In my opinion no one should support this chemical company.

Many everyday household brands use Monsanto's products and should also be avoided at all costs. That brings us to our next chapter. Where are GMO's?

Chapter 3

Where are GMO Foods?

The second step in taking action towards a GMO Free diet is to realize that these genetically altered foods exist everywhere in the United States. Over 50 countries around the world have restrictions or bans on production and sales of GMO foods including all countries in the European Union, Japan and Australia. Despite this they are found everywhere in the U.S. and there are currently no regulations requiring them to be labeled.

Now that you are more aware of what a GMO food is, one would believe these foods should be easy to identify and stay away from, right? That should certainly be the case, but it is far from the truth. It is a discipline that must be practiced regularly with a watchful eye because sadly enough GMO foods are almost everywhere.

There is much obscurity surrounding what is genetically modified and what is not. When you consider the potential risks of consuming these products, knowledge is power.

Our grocery stores are stocked full of GMO foods. Not only must buyer beware of fruits and vegetables, but it is equally important to avoid processed foods. An estimated 70 percent of processed foods on the shelves in our stores contain GMO ingredients, regardless if the product claims to be healthy or not. People trying to eat well or lose weight pick up a box of frozen vegetable burger patties, "healthy soup," or even a "Healthy Choice Meal" only to be putting harmful GM soy and corn into their bodies unknowingly.

There is a common misconception that if something is labeled, "Certified Organic" then it is also non-GMO. This however, is not the case. While it is true that GMOs are excluded under the National Organic Program, GMO testing is not required. "Certified Organic" is required to be at least 95 percent comprised of organic content. The other 5% can be from sources with lower standards and therefore "sneak in" a small amount of GM crops.

Also, organic certification is related to the method of growing the food not about what results from the process. GMO contamination of an "organically grown" product can even occur naturally through cross-pollination, small amounts of genetically modified products occurring in animal food, wind and birds carrying seeds, and from providers of ingredients who might integrate different sources.

The term "GMO food" usually brings to mind fruits, vegetables and beans. Truth is, anything containing genetically modified products that we eat is considered a GMO food. All animal products humans consume that have been fed GMO feed are considered a GMO food. This includes not only meat, but eggs and dairy as well.

The GM industry claims that animals fed genetically modified feed are not in fact genetically modified food products because the genetically modified DNA is broken down completely down in the animals' digestive systems before the consumer even receives the product. This is absolutely untrue.

DNA from genetically modified feed crops was found in milk sold in Italy in 2013, and certainly it existed there before this discovery. Several studies have confirmed genetically modified DNA from feed was taken up by the animals' organs and detected in the meat and fish that people eat, which means it can be passed on to us as we consume it.

The Bt toxin (Bacillus thuringiensis, a soil bacterium used for biological pest control and which has been modified through genetic engineering as previously discussed) is being used in GMO corn and was recently detected in human blood. The UK Government's Food Standards Agency has confirmed that "DNA fragments" of all types in food can be taken up by the digestive tract. "You are what you eat" is a simple truth. Do you know what you are made of?

GMOs are not only found in milk, but also milk products, in forms that could easily go unnoticed. Sometimes, emulsifiers and thickeners are made of GM soybeans and corn. Other times, GM microorganisms produce other additives that are used in dairy products. Some of which are:

Beta-carotene coloring (E 160a); yellow dye used in butter, some dairy desserts, and yogurt.

Riboflavin coloring (E 101: Vitamin B2); used in cheeses and cream products.

Preservatives: Natamycin (E 235), Nisin (E 234), Lysozyme (E 1105); used in cheeses.

Dairy desserts, creams, and puddings sometimes contain emulsifiers and thickeners made from GM soybeans or GM corn.

Egg products also harbor GM ingredients that sometimes fly under the radar. Many mechanically manufactured cream products are made with dried egg powder as opposed to fresh eggs. Two enzymes, lipase and glucose oxidase, are sometimes added to dried egg powder to preserve it and maintain color. These enzymes are produced with the help of GM microorganisms. The same dried egg powder is also sometimes used in pasta and baked goods.

When asking, "Where are GMOs" we also have to consider geographic location. GMOs are labeled, very restricted, or banned in The European Union, Australia, New Zealand, Saudi Arabia, Poland, Brazil, China, Thailand, the Philippines, Fiji, Algeria, Syria, Paraguay, Peru, Japan, Sri Lanka, American Samoa, Cook Islands, Micronesia, Marshall Islands, Nauru, Papua New Guinea, Samoa, Solomon Islands, Tonga, Tuvalu, and Vanuatu.

The United States is home to many large corporations who have a lot of financial interest in the GMO industry. Mistruths that are being fed to the general public have helped to keep US citizens from making too much progress in getting GMOs banned or labeled. The most widely spread mistruth being that GMOs are safe for consumption when there is no scientific evidence to support this claim.

Genetically engineered fish are banned in Maryland. Both North Dakota and Montana are trying to ban genetically engineered wheat. GE crops are banned in Colorado. Mendocino, Marin and Trinity counties in California and San Juan County in Washington State have banned GM crops. Yet there is no guarantee that local and state rulings will be upheld. The Senate recently voted against giving the states the right to inform people of GM foods they are eating with a 71 to 27 vote.

Where are GMO foods? Well, technically almost everywhere. They are found in most parts of the world. Most of the foods in our stores contain them in most of the products that they carry. Most of our animals eat them. From the obvious, to the unsuspecting, the entire planet has been invaded with them. We as individuals must take necessary measures to avoid them at all cost in order to accomplish optimum health.

If you are feeling a little overwhelmed, you are not alone. There are so many potential sources of genetically altered food. But there is hope.

With so many places in the world banning the production and sale of these foods people are obviously having an impact and making their voices heard. Hopefully in my home country of the United States the labeling of these products will soon be mandatory at the very least. After all, if you are going to take part in an experiment involving your body, wouldn't you like to know?

I like to keep things simple in my life. The fact that so much money is spent by GMO food companies to prevent the labeling of these foods is proof enough for me that these companies know the foods they produce are potentially dangerous at the very least.

So we are now at a crossroads. Deciding whether or not to take place in this experiment is a decision that we must all make for ourselves. Some choose to simply ignore this issue and go on with their lives paying no attention to what they ingest or the companies they support. These individuals don't worry or care where their food comes from or its ingredients, and instead focus on the price and flavor of a food.

People who actively pursue their health and well being do not behave this way. This group of individuals wants to make educated decisions and take focused action to insure their own personal health as much as possible.

We all have the power of choice. Which group would you like to belong to?

Chapter 4

The Top 10 Genetically Modified Foods

The next action step in the GMO Free Diet is to identify the most common sources of GMO food and make sure you acquire these items from a trusted source or simply eliminate them. In this chapter, we will cover the top 10 GM foods most widely available for purchase. Obviously this list is only the tip of the iceberg. A large portion of this list are foods that are used to make a wide range of different foods and products, so staying away from them is key to staying on track and eating healthy and well.

1. Corn

Most everyone has heard about GMO corn. Half of the US farms growing corn are growing GMO corn. The largest portion of this corn is intended for human consumption. This same corn has been known to cause weight gain and organ disruption. Mice fed GMO corn were found to not only develop cancer, but have reproductive problems and smaller offspring as well. Corn products are everywhere and include foods that contain corn oil, corn starch, corn flour, and high fructose corn syrup.

2. Soy

As much as 90% of soybeans in the market have been altered to be resistant to herbicides, specifically Monsanto's Roundup. In 2006, soybeans in the U.S. were sprayed with 96.7 million pounds of glyphosate (Roundup). Not only is soy a GMO food, it is undoubtedly full of chemicals. Hamsters that ate GMO soy had a very high mortality rate and were incapable of reproducing. Soy is found in tofu, soybean oil, soy flour, soy beverages, and other products such as baked goods, vegetarian foods and pastries.

3. Canola/Rapeseed
Canola oil is derived from rapeseed; Canada named it canola so it would not be confused with the non-edible rapeseed. It is used in cooking oil and margarine. One third of honey in Canada was discovered to contain GM rapeseed pollen.

4. Cotton
GMO cotton is altered to increase harvest and be resistant to disease. Cotton from India and China are the highest risk. Why is cotton on the list? Cotton is not a food is it? No but it is one of the most commonly grown GM crops and purchasing genetically modified cotton only contributes to the problem at hand. Invest a little time to research your purchases involving cotton and select sources that do not use GM cotton. Money is after all a very powerful vote and we do not want to support these companies or their purpose.

5. Milk and Dairy Products

Dairy products are full of growth hormones. One fifth of the cows in the U.S. are treated with hormones which speed their growth and increase the amount of milk they can produce. These hormones have been shown to have an adverse effect on the human body. Monsanto's rBGH is still in most US cows but is oddly enough banned in 27 other countries. Not to mention that most livestock in the US is fed GM feed.

6. Sugar

GM sugar beets resistant to Roundup showed up in the U.S. in 2009. There are many alternatives to sugar. Some natural ones that come to mind are agave nectar and honey. When using sweeteners, whatever you use, don't use number 7 on this list.

7. Aspartame

Aspartame is a toxic sugar substitute made from genetically modified bacteria. There is major concern that it has major harmful effects on the human body including cancer. It is very controversial and is hiding everywhere. Make sure it is not in your kitchen.

8. Zucchini

Genetically modified zucchini has a toxic protein that acts as an insecticide. It has been found in the blood of humans, most disturbingly in that of pregnant women and their fetuses. I love vegetables and especially zucchini, but a little extra time must be taken to make sure that your zucchini is not from genetically modified crop.

9. Yellow squash

Yellow squash has the same genetic modifications as zucchini.

10. Papaya

Papayas have been genetically modified and grown in Hawaii since 1999. The papayas are slow to mature and resistant to the Papaya Ringspot virus. Papayas are less commonly consumed in the US but if you do eat papaya then make sure it is not GM.

A list of ten looks short, but the amount of byproducts produced by these crops is a much lengthier one. GM feed is fed to animals that we not only eat directly but we also consume byproducts made from their milk and eggs. This is how GMOs remain abundant in products like ice cream, cheese, mayo, veggie burgers, and even whey protein. There are thousands of processed foods out there and GMOs are used in many, from infant formula to tofu, tortillas, and marinara sauce.

The health hazards of some of these foods are well-publicized. DNA from genetically modified crops has already been detected in human beings. There is absolutely no way to know what dangerous effects these lab-modified foods will have on our future health.

For a moment, think about all the health risks that are still undiscovered. Due to the current lack of regulation and safety measures taken by those in the GMO industry, there is no possible way to know what other risks these lab-created foods pose to us.

Again this is not meant to overwhelm. A GMO Free Diet can be achieved. Educating yourself on the most common GMO's and developing a game plan is what we are trying to accomplish. This brings us to our next chapter, some of the specific companies involved.

Chapter 5

Companies that use Genetically Modified Ingredients

The next critical action step that must be taken in avoiding GMO foods is to identify the companies that promote their use by using GMOs in their products. Knowing which companies regularly use GMO ingredients and products can be an immensely useful weapon in fighting the battle to eliminate these foods. Most products sold as "health foods" and "natural foods" in your local grocery store are not healthy or natural by any stretch of the imagination.

If these companies will use GM ingredients in some of their products (especially those marketed as healthy) you can rest assured that they use it in most, if not all, of what they produce.

Many large corporations use GMO ingredients, big surprise. Many consumers are unaware that these large corporations buy up and own smaller companies and use the same ingredients. The smaller company brands are often the ones marketed as healthy and natural. The average consumer does not always recognize this tactic and is unable to make well-informed purchases. Consider yourself informed.

Here are just a few:

Act II (popcorn), Aunt Jemima, Aurora Foods, Baker's, Banquet, Bearnaise, Beech-nut, Bestfoods, Betty Crocker, Bertoli, Bird's, Bisquik, Blue Sky, Boca, Budget Gourmet, Cadbury, Capri Sun, Carnation, Celeste, Coca Cola, Con Agra, Country Inn Specialties, Chef Boyardee, Dannon, Del Monte, Delicious Brands, Dinty Moore, Duncan Hines, Eggo, Enfamil, Five Brothers Pasta Sauce, Famous Amos, Flowers Industries, Franco-American, Frito-Lay, Frookies, Fruitopia, Fruit works, Gatorade, General Mills, Good Start, Green Giant, Hansen, Hawaiian Punch, Healthy Choice, Heinz Products, Hellman's, Hershey's, Hi-C, Holsum, Hormel, Hungry Jack, Hunt's, Interstate Bakeries, Isomil, Keebler, Kellogs, Kid Cuisine, Kids' Kitchen, Koolaid, Knorr, Kraft, Land-o-Lakes, Libby's, Lipton, Lean Cuisine, Loma Linda, Marie Callendar's, Morningstar Farms,

Mrs Butterworths, Nabisco, Natural Touch, Near East, Nestle, Nutra Blend Soy, Ocean Spray, Ore-Ida, Ortega, Orville Redenbacher, Parmalat, Pasta Sauce Packets Alfredo, Pasta Roni, Pepperidge Farm, Pepsi Co, Phillip Morris, Pillsbury, Pop Secret, Post, Power Bar, Pringles, Prego, Procter & Gamble, Progresso, Quaker, Ragu, Red Oval Farms, Rice-a-Roni, Rosetto Frozen Pasta, Sesame Street, Snack Wells, Similac, Skippy, Smuckers, Stouffers, Sunshine, Swanson, Swiss Miss, Thomas', Tombstone, Tostito's Salsa, Totino's, Tropicana, Uncle Ben's, Unilever, V-8, Viola!, Weight Watchers, Wonder, Worthington, and Yoplait.

The truth is the amount of companies using GMO ingredients is too large to list in this book. In actuality, there is no complete index of manufacturers that use GMO foods. This list was included so you would recognize the everyday household brands and realize that these products are everywhere.

Research and knowledge of the foods themselves, along with information on the companies that you purchase your food from is essential.

It has become an unfortunate but necessary truth that you must actually research where your food is coming from.

Because this books main focus is on genetically modified ingredients and not one specific type of diet, it would be inefficient and irrelevant to try and list the things that should and should not be eaten on this diet. The focus is eating food that has not been genetically modified.

Some are vegans while others are meat eaters. People trying to lose weight are obviously going to have a different caloric requirement than someone training for an athletic event.

For specific dieting information please refer to the recommended reading in the back of this book.

Whatever kind of diet you subscribe to, the method I describe in chapter 6 for eating a diet completely free of GMO's will work for anyone. This is the method I use and not only does it work for weeding out the dangerous foods and food additives; it also will save you a ton of money.

.

Chapter 6

Myths and Truths about GMO Foods

There is much controversy surrounding GM foods. The general public receives information that is passed down from the biotech industry and government supporters. Because regulation of GM foods is relaxed in the US and Canada compared to regulations in European countries, most North Americans are oblivious to the fact that they are being used as lab rats. This is partially due to the fact that manufacturers are not required to label their products. Profit is the goal and both technology and agriculture are being heavily invested in because agriculture is a huge export in the US.

The result is the mass majority of North Americans living in the dark in regard to what they are really eating. This chapter is devoted to shedding light on a few of the myths surrounding GM foods.

Myth 1: GM foods are regulated by the FDA and other agencies for the safety of US citizens.

The Truth: The regulation of GM foods ranges from very lenient in most of the world to non-existent in the United States. In 1990 the FDA pulled rank on its own scientists and formed their own GM policy requiring absolutely no labeling or safety testing.

Myth 2: Human consumption of GM foods is safe.

The Truth: GM foods can be unpredictably toxic and/or allergenic. This is because the placement of genes from one species to another results in a very unpredictable substance. Numerous studies have found severe damaging effects on the health of mice, rats and livestock who ate GMO feed. In one study 93 per cent of blood taken from expecting women, and 80 percent from umbilical, came up positive for toxins acquired from GMO foods that they had eaten. Glyphosate (Roundup) and Gluphosinate (an herbicide) have both been found in the bloodstreams of non-pregnant women as well.

One can only guess how many dangerous side-effects will show themselves in years to come as the consumption of GM foods is still a relatively new practice.

Myth 3: GM Bt insecticidal crops harm only insects and are harmless to those who eat them.

The Truth: This statement assumes that natural Bt and GM Bt are the same and this is untrue. Bt in natural form comes from a bacteria found in soil. There has been at least a 40% difference found between the natural and GM Bt insecticides. Bt insecticidal crops have been found to be toxic for many organs in the digestive system and disruptive of the immune systems in animals who have digested such feed.

Findings include toxic effects on the small intestine, liver, kidney, spleen, pancreas, and disturbances in the digestive and immune systems of the animals that eat them. The GM Bt protein is expressed in every cell of the plant, so therefore the plant becomes an insecticide. We can deduce then that the person or animal eating it becomes such as well.

Myth 4: GM crops increase yield potential.

The Truth: GM crops have not increased yield potential. In many cases yield has decreased. Genetically modified crops have shown no greater yield than non-GM crops. Genetically modified soybeans have been producing even lower yields. Studies comparing GM and non-GM soy crops suggested that 50% of the drop is triggered by disruption in genes due to the genetic modification method. Tests of Bt corn showed that they actually produced up to 12% less yields and took longer to mature than non-GM corn. A USDA report highlights the poor yielding of genetically modified crops, stating, "GE [genetically engineered] crops available for commercial use do not increase the yield potential of a variety.

In fact, yield may even decrease...."
Perhaps the biggest issue raised by
these results is how to explain the
rapid adoption of GE crops, when
farm financial results appear to be
mixed or even negative."

Myth 5: GM crops decrease the
use of pesticide.

The Truth: GM crops have had a
huge increase in pesticide
(including herbicide) use. Since
1996, GM crops increased the use
of pesticide by 383 million pounds.
This is due to the fact that weeds
are now becoming herbicide-
resistant "superweeds." Farmers
have to use more toxic herbicides
than before and Monsanto happily
provides them with an endless
supply. All part of the plan I'm
sure.

Myth 6: GM crops are "environmentally friendly" because they are considered "no-till" farming.

The Truth: In this case the negative effects completely outweigh the positive. Sure, GM crops may be "no-till," but we have effectively increased the amount of toxic chemicals released into the environment while simultaneously creating a new breed of "superweed" that is resistant to "safe" herbicide.

Myth 7: Monsanto's glyphosate, known as Roundup, is a nonthreatening, biodegradable herbicide.

The Truth: Roundup was forced to remove the term biodegradable from its packaging. Roundup persists in the environment and has toxic effects on wildlife. During crop growing season, the toxin known as Roundup was found in 60-100% of air and rain samples taken from the Midwest. Yuck.

Myth 8: GM and Non-GM crops have the ability to coexist.

The Truth: This claim is very far from the truth. Natural cross-pollination is producing small amounts of GMO DNA in Non GMO crops today! Wind and birds carrying seeds have led to extensive contamination of both organic and non-GM crops.

Myth 9: GM crops are essential to feed the increasing population.

The Truth: The answer to feeding the world's growing population has nothing to do with GM crops. Genetically modified crops simply do not deliver higher yields than non-GM crops. Hunger is a problem of distribution and poverty. Growing genetically modified crops in poor countries is making this problem even worse. Let's examine the "terminator" seed technology. This seed is genetically altered to grow only one season and produce non viable seeds from the harvest. In effect this forces a population to purchase a new batch of seeds only good for the one growing season, and the cycle then repeats. This obviously is not designed to feed the population of the world, but to consolidate wealth to the seed patent holders.

Myth 10: GM crops are instrumental in attaining food security.

The Truth: The answer does not lie in the genetics of the plants or animals, it lays in the way that crops and animals are grown and raised. By using sustainable farming methods that preserve soil and water and reduce external inputs, we can not only ensure that there is enough food for the current population, but that the land stays productive for future generations. We can make sure there is enough food for current and future generations by coming up with and putting into practice sustainable farming methods that reduce external inputs and preserve soil and water.

Chapter 7

How to Avoid GMO Foods

This next step in sustaining a GMO free diet is an obvious one. To completely abstain from consuming any product that contains GMO's in any form as much as possible. We have only covered the surface of genetically modified foods. This topic goes very deep and can be studied in great detail, but hopefully you now understand that these foods are dangerous. They are artificially created and full of genetic mutations that have already been detected in human blood.

When you stop and think about all the disorders and diseases humans are faced with today, these foods are definitely not helping anyone sleep better at night.

Let's get started with some basic guidelines:

1. Never purchase corn and soy products that are not clearly branded as 100% Organic. Remember that 88% of corn is GMO and soy is even higher at 93%. Foods labeled as 100 % organic cannot contain any genetically modified organisms according to the USDA Organic Program standards.

   It would be an ever better idea to nix these two products from your diet completely as even something labeled "Certified Organic" only technically has to be 95%. If it does not say it is 100% organic then it is probably a combination of ingredients. Do not forget that processed foods usually contain some byproduct of corn or soy, so steer clear of them completely whenever possible.

2. A useful tool in shopping for non-GMO fruits and vegetables are PLU (Price Look Up) codes that are located on most produce in the form of a sticker, stamp, or label. Retailers use these codes to ring up bulk produce items. The codes identify exactly what the item is with its current pricing, while giving the consumer a handy tag for identifying GMO produce.

Packaged produce or items that are too small to label or stamp do not usually have the PLU visible. PLU codes contain five digits. The key is to look at the first digit. If it is a 9, the item is organic.

If it is an 8, it is definitely a GMO. Conventionally grown produce has a 0 for the first digit but it is usually left off so it appears to be only four digits.

3. A good rule of thumb is to buy organic from local farmers at farmer's markets and local health food stores. By going this route it is easier to find out exactly how these products were raised. Also, purchase items that may not necessarily be convenient like bulk dried organic beans and lentils.

4. Organic gardening is always a good option for getting non-GMO produce. What better way to enjoy the literal fruits of your labor!? It can be hard work, but it will pay off in more ways than one. It is a sure fire way to know where and how your produce is

grown. Be sure to get your seeds from a trusted source. Check out the suggested reading in the back of the book to help make this endeavor a little easier should you decide to go this route.

The method I personally use saves me time, money, and I believe will work for anyone that has just an hour or two to dedicate to the process.

The method involves sitting down with a piece of paper and investing a small amount of time to write down your specific chosen meals that you will eat that week or month. You can choose these meals based on your specific health or fitness goal. Some opt out of carbohydrate consumption (no carb or slow carb diet), others only eat raw ingredients (raw food diet).

Next you will prepare a shopping list and include all of the ingredients you need to prepare your dishes. I actually use the same recipe for most of my meals as I have found that eating the same meals over and over again help me to stick to my diet plan and control my appetite. I find something I like and I run with it. When you choose dishes you like and that taste good to you, I have found it is easier to follow the lifestyle design plan that you have chosen.

The list you have prepared is now ready to be researched. Again choose meals that will nourish your specific health goal and that taste great for you. Some will choose a goal of weight loss, others a high protein and high calorie goal for athletic training. Invest an hour or two of your time to research where you can obtain these ingredients from a local trusted source. You can do this research yourself, or use a trusted resource such as a personal trainer or diet coach to locate the ingredients you need to prepare your meals.

In the back of the book I provide some very useful resources for researching your shopping list yourself as well as some suggestions for common items that are non GMO.

This research only needs to be done periodically and you can use the same sources again and again. Your research should be checked every so often as many small food producers have been bought by larger corporations and then continued to be marketed to the public as healthy. If you eat beef, search out beef that has been fed organically raised feed or grown by a local rancher that you can trust. If you are a vegetarian, likewise search out vegetables grown 100% organic from non genetically modified seeds.

This may sound like common sense and guess what, it is. However the majority of people do not take this critical step. They begin their diet of salads and whole foods with the intention of becoming more fit and healthy and in reality are gambling with their health. Why take this chance? Are you really that busy? Considering the alternative, this step is a must.

Fortunately there are many products available today that do label their products as Non GMO because they realize that there is a demand for these products. This is great news for those of us seeking these kinds of products.

To make this whole process easier, as I have stated before, continue to purchase the same ingredients from the same trusted sources as much as possible. This eliminates the need for constantly wondering if what you are eating is safe.

I personally start my day almost every day with a 100% Organic plant based protein drink that you can mix with water. No blending required. One serving of this Non GMO product is equal to 24 servings of vegetables and is great for alkalizing your system. Wheat grass is also another great option. Check the resources section for details.

I also recommend putting together a list of fun foods and researching them in a similar fashion. Some deserts and cheat day foods should be thought out because we all break the rules sometime. So prepare for this by not running out and buying an impulse food. Instead have some foods available that have already been researched and you can easily access them on those rainy days. Some examples of this could be a homemade recipe for ice cream using pure ingredients or a simple fruit smoothie.

In addition I have a list of travel foods. For me this list is narrow. I try to only purchase certified organic foods while on the road from local farmer markets and shop market chains that carry organic products.

Obviously eating on the road is easier when eating a raw food diet. If you are a meat eater or like to eat hot foods I suggest bringing a small camp stove and pan.

Of course depending on the length of your trip you can always prepare some meals in advance. I myself have equipped my truck with a small cook kit. I keep a gallon of water for cleanup and eat healthy on the go. This is accomplished using standard kitchen equipment, a container to store the equipment in your vehicle, and an off the shelf power inverter that plugs into the cigarette lighter of your vehicle or hooks directly to the vehicles battery. I am a believer in using the resources you have available to you.

For instant smoothies I keep a small blender in the vehicle. These smoothies are often $5 or more at the local juice bar depending on where you live, and you usually have no knowledge of the ingredients being used. In the resources section at the end of this book there are some helpful links for setting up a travelling cook station. This will not only save you a fortune but is by far the healthiest way to eat in my opinion because you are controlling all ingredients.

This can be a tough discipline to master. For most, they believe they are just too busy and would rather drive through a fast food restaurant.

While this may sound odd to some, it saves you a ton of money when you stop visiting fast food chains and restaurants, and you can make whatever you want instead of having to choose from a menu. It is actually easier than you think to get into this habit. You just make what you want right on the spot. You don't have to wait to go camping to cook outside. You can cook a quick meal, cleanup and be on your way in just minutes. Don't believe me? Sound like too much work? I do it all the time and I promise you it's not that hard.

Obviously the less you have to prepare a meal the more convenient it becomes. Raw diets are ideal for travelling because they require no cooking at all.

Don't like to make your own food? Don't worry this diet can still work for you. There are a variety of frozen foods on the market these days that are non GMO. If just popping something in the oven is more your style, then there are options for you as well. I personally believe you should get in the habit of making your own food, but don't let this discourage you if you are just starting on your path towards health. Making small changes to your diet over time is beneficial as long as you stick with it.

One item I have found extremely helpful are the Organic live food bars available from the Raw Revolution Organic Company. These are made with Non GMO ingredients and are loaded with vitamins and protein from real food.

They are also great for eating on the run and snacking when you can't really get a meal in. These are available at many health food stores and supermarkets, or you can check the resources section of this book for where these delicious snacks are sold specifically.

I must acknowledge that we all have our weaknesses. There are times when ingesting these foods is bound to happen. This is a common problem for all diets, and like all other diets, the key is not to beat one's self up over the occasional indulgence. Instead, realize that you are minimizing your consumption of these items and carry on from this positive perspective.

The main principals to focus on are:

1. Eat whole foods and avoid all processed foods. If you wish to consume processed foods I recommend investing in a food processor and renewing the lost art of making your own food from known and trusted ingredients.
2. Eat foods that are labeled 100% Organic or Non-GMO.
3. Take the time to create a researched shopping list of all ingredients used in your recipes.
4. Support trusted local sources of food when at all possible.
5. Have a plan for eating on the go. Due your localized research and know the markets and cafes around you that you carry or prepare Non GMO foods.

6. Do not support companies that are making this a difficult lifestyle choice in the first place. Ideally we would not like to worry about this problem at all. But the threat is there and very real. Not supporting these companies could lead to the end of these foods in circulation, at which point the advice in this book would become joyfully obsolete.

Fruits, vegetables and natural foods have never posed a risk in the past. Unfortunately that is no longer the case.

Exercise your power of choice. Businesses cater to the customer so ask for Non GMO foods often. Force restaurants and grocery markets to respond to the demand for REAL food.

You must remember that every dish you have ever eaten can be prepared using 100% real foods as opposed to GM food. Even the meals that we think of as unhealthy or indulgent would be less damaging if prepared using Non GMO ingredients.

A diet is not something you do for a short period of time to get the body you want overnight. A diet is a lifestyle design and you want to create a design that is healthy and enjoyable. Free of disease and ailments.

Maintaining a GMO Free Diet is work. Like any diet it is practice and discipline. It requires knowledge, a watchful eye, and a bit of footwork, but it is a priceless venture.

Please visit my website at www.NewSustainableLiving.com today and stay current on all the latest sustainable living news and events.

Conclusion

Thank you again for reading this book!

I hope this book was able to help you to create a diet free from GMO ingredients.

If you enjoyed this book, please take the time to share your thoughts and post a review on Amazon. It would be greatly appreciated!

As a thank you for your purchase of this book,

Digital Direct Publishing would like to offer you a FREE subscription to our FREE eBook Newsletter. Everyone loves a good read, especially when it's free. We offer select titles to our subscribers free of charge every day. Go to www.Digital Direct Publishing.com and signup.

Thank you and good luck towards your goals!

Resources

When it comes to avoiding genetically modified foods, especially in the United States, having some simple systems in place is a good idea. As promised here are some of the resources I use as well as some recommended documentaries and books.

If you are interested in self sustainability and the art of living healthy and financially free, please subscribe to my blog here or go to NewSustainableLiving.com for valuable information on topics from shelter construction to organic gardening.

Recommended Documentaries:

The World According to Monsanto Directed by Marie-Monique Robin

Genetic Roulette: The Gamble of Our Lives
Jeffrey M. Smith (Director)

Both of these documentaries are very informative and well done in my opinion. Please support the filmmakers by visiting the website and ordering these titles.

Recommended Reading:

Here are a couple of great books that cover some more healthy eating techniques.

How to Lose Massive Weight with the Alkaline Diet.
By Ma Rose

The Juicing Bible by Pat Crocker

Recommended Non GMO Products:

Raw Revolution Organic Live Food Bars

I eat these all the time during my busy days. No matter how big of a hurry you find yourself in, these snacks are tasty, healthy, and Non GMO.

Spirulina Dream is my favorite of these but there are many flavors to choose from.

GMO Free Garbanzo Beans | 100% USA Grown | Identity Preserved (We Tell You Which Farm We Grew It In) | 5 Lbs

The Palouse Brand is a great source for all of the essentials. When buying food from this company you are guaranteed Non GMO whole foods. Run by the Mader Family for five generations and located in Southeast Washington state, they not only supply a variety of Non GMO foods, they also label every bag of food with the exact farm where it was produced. They also have <u>Wheat Berries</u>, <u>Lentils</u>, <u>Split Peas</u> and more.

Tiny But Mighty Heirloom Popcorn ~ virtually hulless Non-GMO popping corn
With GM Corn being one of the largest GMO crops out there, here is a great choice for the folks that just want to relax with a bowl of popcorn.

Lemon Poppy Seed Muffin Mixes Organic, Non-GMO. These muffin mixes are great for the people that like to bake. You will also be avoiding GMO's baking with these mixes.

I have to mention what I drink in the morning for breakfast that makes me feel great. It is a plant based protein drink that is equivalent to 24 servings of vegetables. I found this on the shelf at a local health food store a couple years ago and really have been drinking it ever since.

First thing in the morning, when my body craves water, I drink a tall glass of this green drink. It hydrates, alkalizes the blood, and there is 25 grams of plant based proteins as well.

Paradise Herbs Energy Protein Powder Greens
is reasonably priced and just mixes with water so you can bring it with you and drink it anywhere. For the athletes and active people reading, it aids in muscle recovery much like your standard post workout protein drink, but this drink is Non GMO.

If I don't have the protein greens I go for some fresh juice or lemon water. Always opting for drinking water without fluoride.

Recommended Kitchen and Cooking Equipment:

If you want to cook from scratch with healthy ingredients a food processor is an awesome tool. For making everything from salsa to nut butters, these are definitely useful pieces of technology.

The Cuisinart DLC-10S Pro Classic 7-Cup Food Processor works really well and isn't too expensive for how long they last.

I really like drinking fresh juice of all kinds but especially a carrot, tomato, and cucumber blend. If you have not tried it, a V8 vegetable juice is no comparison. For me it feels like drinking from the fountain of youth. I really feel energized and ready to get something done after a tall glass of fresh made juice.

The Breville JE98XL Juice Fountain Plus 850-Watt Juice Extractor is the juicer I use. I have had it for a good long while now and I use it everyday a couple of times a day. It is easy to clean up as long as you get to it within a few minutes of finishing your juicing. One thing about juicing I have found is that it's real easy to clean the machine when you do it right away. If you let it sit around on the counter or in the sink it becomes more of a chore than necessary to clean up.

Recommended Travel Supplies:

If you want to be able to just make a fresh smoothie from pretty much anywhere then you will want to use a **NutriBullet**.

You can use these on the road after popping into a market and getting some fresh Organic Produce. Just pour some water in when finished and give it a couple shakes for an easy cleanup when you get home.

For those of you like me that like to save money over the long term by investing in the right equipment up front, then you will want to pick up a **Cobra 2500 Watt Power Inverter**

This inverter will power any kitchen appliance you can think of. If you own a vehicle you are literally driving around in a portable power station. Why not put it to good use?

At $5 or more for a smoothie at a health food store or juice bar, it won't take long for this equipment to pay for itself.

I am here to help. If you are having trouble finding a particular Non GMO product in your area or for more information about anything in this book, please contact me through my website at www.NewSustainableLiving.com.

Thank you and I hope you achieve all of your healthy lifestyle goals.

Made in the USA
San Bernardino, CA
30 March 2014